I0759219

Type 2 Diabetes Diagnosis and Complications

Control the Mental and Physical Challenges of Receiving This Potentially Debilitating Diagnosis

Ron Kness

No part of this book may be reproduced, stored in a retrieval system, or transmitted in any form or by any means, electronic, mechanical, photocopying, recording, scanning, or otherwise, without the prior written permission of the publisher, except for the inclusion of brief quotations in a review.

This book is for **personal use only**.

Published by:

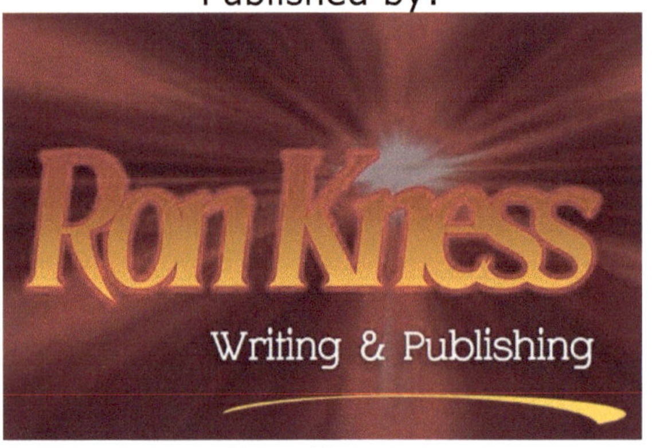

Ron Kness

San Tan Valley, AZ

United States of America

ISBN: 9781798192153

Copyright © 2019 – Ron Kness – All Rights Reserved

Contents

Introduction

Being told that you have Type 2 diabetes is an often a shocking and depressing diagnosis. Everyone reacts differently to being told they have the disease. There are those who brush it off as nothing, and those who assume it means their entire life will be upended.

The reality is, you can safely live a normal and happy life if you understand how your body reacts to food, stress, exercise and other lifestyle factors (like sleep), and educate yourself for health and safety.

One of the reasons people get so upset is that there's a lot of information to learn when it comes to managing your diabetes. But it doesn't have to all be digested and understood in one day.

Throughout this book, I have highlighted words that can take you to more information about controlling Type 2 diabetes or a related topic. To get to that information, go to the Resources page toward the end of this book and to the link next to the word that was highlighted. I have arranged all the words and their respective links according to chapter titles.

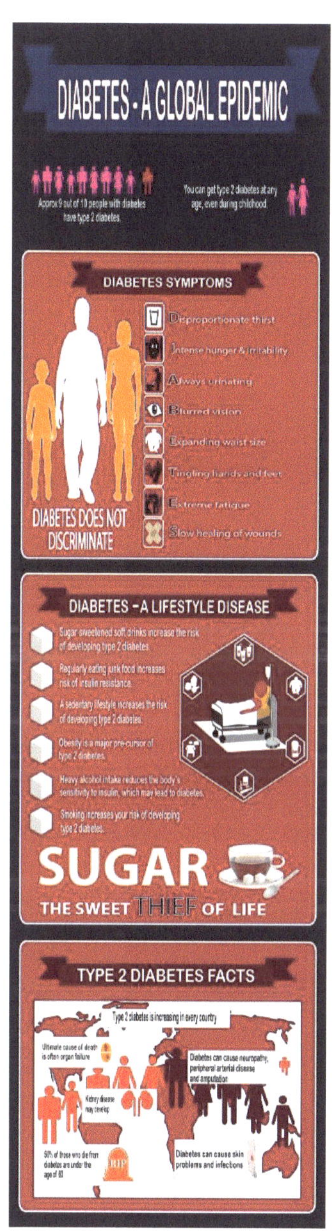

I have a whole website devoted to Diabetes Management. The blog posts are free for you to read, some information is free to download, and I have an information store where you can purchase additional information on diabetes at reasonable prices if you want to, along with some books published on Amazon on diabetes and related topics. You will find links to these sites in the Resources page.

Controlling diabetes is a lifelong process, and you'll be discovering things along the way that help you feel better and react better to things going on in your life. Yes, food is a huge component of what you must learn.

The nutrition you consume can either worsen or improve your diabetes diagnosis. But it's not the only factor contributing to or helping the disease. Other things are equally important.

For example, if you have chronic stress in your life, the cortisol (stress hormone) coursing through your body will have a negative impact on your blood sugar levels. Likewise, a lack of sleep impairs the body's ability to recover and support you properly with this condition.

This disease isn't one where you'll be perfect 24 hours a day, 365 days a year. There will be times when you do something that doesn't help your diagnosis. The key is in how you effectively manage the disease over long periods of time.

The worst thing you can do is assume diabetes is nothing more than an inconvenience with food, because it's much more than a disease that makes you feel a bit "off" here and there.

It can cause major problems with your eyesight, limbs, and it can even be fatal if left unmanaged, so you need to grasp the various ways a Type 2 diabetes diagnosis can affect every aspect of your body.

Aside from learning how to manage the condition and how certain things affect you personally, you'll want to understand how diabetes worsens the body so you can be alert for signs and symptoms of problems that might arise.

Type 2 Diabetes and Your Heart

Research has shown that one of the organs greatly impacted by diabetes is the heart. The statistics for cardiac or heart-related disease among those with diabetes is astounding.

Nearly 70% of people with diabetes have died from a heart-related event. If you have the disease, your risk of dying from a heart attack or heart disease is quadruple what the statistics show for people who don't have the condition.

Why the Heart Suffers When You Have Diabetes

There's no doubt that diabetes is a difficult disease. It can make you feel bad physically and emotionally. The fact that there is no cure for the condition makes many people feel like there's no hope.

But as with many diseases, diabetes is completely manageable, and you should try your best to do exactly that. People who don't keep their diabetes under control are more likely to have a heart attack or heart disease than diabetics that do practice good lifestyle habits.

However, just having the disease alone is enough to greatly raise your risk factor. There are several reasons why you're likely to have problems with your heart if you have diabetes.

People with diabetes usually have higher than healthy levels of cholesterol. High cholesterol means that your blood flow can eventually become restricted due to cholesterol building up plaque within your blood vessels.

When the arteries become narrowed from the buildup, your heart is impacted from lack of proper blood flow. So it has to work harder to pump - and to keep you alive - but it can't overcome arteries that reach the stage where not enough blood gets through.

High cholesterol can be an inherited trait. For people with diabetes, this trait can be worsened by bad habits such as not eating healthy, not exercising and carrying too much weight.

But just because you're at a higher risk doesn't mean that achieving good health is hopeless. Cholesterol can be lowered if you practice smart health habits. You can take control and change those levels just as you can every other aspect of your daily life that can negatively impact your heart because of diabetes.

One of these wise habits to implement is exercise. Not exercising can impact your heart. If you're not physically active and you don't have diabetes, it can hurt your heart health - but not to the same degree or with the same risks involved as when you do have it.

The reason that not exercising causes heart issues for diabetics is because exercise is one the best ways to eliminate glucose from the bloodstream. Being physically active helps your body process glucose and fights back against insulin resistance.

Plus, engaging in the right kind of exercise lowers your chances of having a heart attack. If you can, you should commit to a regular regimen involving aerobic exercise - but if you can't, then even getting up and moving more can help.

Anything that makes you sweat can improve your body's ability to use glucose and helps lower the risk for your heart. Even if you can only exercise 15 to 20 minutes a day, that does a lot to strengthen and protect your heart.

The Four Steps You Can Take to Lower Your Risk of Heart Problems

When it comes to diabetes, it's not hopeless. While you may not be able to roll the clock back in time and take away the diagnosis, you *can* live in such a way that you're healthier from here on out.

When you do that, your heart won't face the same level of damage, if any. The very first thing you need to do when you've been told you have diabetes is to take stock of your weight.

You may or may not be obese when you get the diagnosis. But if you are obese, your risk factor jumps to the top of the chart. It's one of the most common factors involved in heart related incidents such as heart attacks.

Carrying around too much excess weight prohibits your body from being able to use insulin correctly. Regardless of whether your body is still making some or you must go on insulin shots, your weight can be the leading cause of insulin resistance.

When you lose weight, your body becomes more sensitive to insulin. - because then it's able to better use the glucose and you end up lowering your risks of heart health problems.

The second step you can take is to get your blood pressure under control. Losing weight if you're obese will naturally help to lower it. But in the meantime, while it's still high, it can be causing damage to heart.

High blood pressure is one of the main causes of heart attacks. It happens because the higher your blood pressure, the greater the strain on your heart. Having high blood pressure causes damage to the arteries giving blood to your heart.

By taking medication, losing weight and exercising, you can greatly reduce the impact to your heart. The third step you need to take is to stop smoking if you currently do. Smoking increases your risk of developing heart problems.

When smoking is coupled with diabetes, heart attacks and damage are more common. Finally, the fourth step and the number one reason your heart is heavily impacted by disease is because of glucose levels that are consistently out of control.

When you have diabetes, your glucose can elevate to the point that not only does it damage your heart, causing heart disease - but it can also be fatal. Medications for diabetes can only do so much to keep your levels within a normal range.

If you sabotage the effects of the medication with poor lifestyle choices, then you're gambling with the health of your heart. Those are stakes that are just too high. The longer your levels are out of range, the more damage that's being done to your blood vessels and ultimately your heart.

There are specific heart-healthy diet plans that can double as heart-friendly nutritional guidance as well as weight loss plans. There are several plans that promote heart health as well as weight loss – you just must choose which one works best for you.

The [Mediterranean Diet](#) is perfect for those who have diabetes and want to lose weight and protect their heart. You'll want to modify the diet so that it's best for diabetics, but you'll enjoy diabetic relief from parts of the program, such as enjoying lean meat and healthy product while avoiding high doses of sugar and other carbs.

The Ornish Diet is another heart-healthy plan. It's low in saturated fat and cholesterol foods as well as carbs, making it a great prospect for diabetics. If carbs are included, they're complex carbs, so you'll want to see how your body responds to that. This plan also emphasizes good lifestyle habits, such as stress management, smoking cessation and other beneficial changes.

The DASH Diet might be a good choice for you as a diabetic who wants to protect his or her heart. However, you'll want to watch the inclusion of carbs carefully. It allows for fruits and grains, but also emphasizes lean proteins with an avoidance of saturated fats and high sugar content foods.

The MIND Diet was initially planned for diseases like Alzheimer's, but the focus on leafy greens, nuts and other vegetables along with fish and poultry make this a diet designed perfectly for diabetics.

Take a multi-pronged approach to your heart health as a diabetic and you'll prevent a lot of damage that might otherwise occur with this disease. From nutrition to exercise to stress relief, you can manage the condition and protect your heart and other organs easily.

Diabetics Have an Increased Risk of Stroke

You may already know many of the side effects of living with diabetes. One side effect of having the disease puts you at a higher risk of having a stroke at some point in your life.

While just having the disease alone is enough to make you more vulnerable to this health event, for those who don't control their diabetes, it's much worse. People who don't keep their glucose levels managed will have a higher chance of having a stroke.

When your blood sugar is consistently high, it can lead to problems with your blood vessels. What happens is that as you continually subject your vessels to the elevated glucose, it causes plaque to develop.

At the first development of plaque, you won't notice any symptoms and you won't have any issues. But as time passes, this plaque gets thicker. Over time, it adheres to the inside of your blood vessels and can cause narrowed passages.

This means that the way your blood normally travels through the area is now altered because it's thinner. So your blood has to try to get through passages that don't have enough room.

When the vessels get blocked to a certain point, the result causes a stroke to happen. A stroke shuts off the blood supply to your brain. It does this by creating a blockage such as with a clot or by causing a blood vessel to rupture.

The stroke then affects whichever part of the brain where it occurred. This is why some people, after suffering from a stroke, have trouble speaking or walking or doing other things they normally would do.

The most worrisome problem with being a diabetic with a stroke risk is that, unlike certain diseases you might get, a stroke doesn't let you know that it's on the way. One minute you're feeling fine and then next, you're in the middle of having the stroke.

The longer you go untreated after having a stroke, the more you'll experience physical side effects from the event. There are several reasons why diabetes can increase your risk of stroke.

Your genetics play a role in whether or not your risk is elevated. Not having your blood pressure under control can also lead to a stroke. When your blood pressure is elevated, it puts more pressure on your heart.

It must expend more energy than it would if your blood pressure was within s normal range. In fact, the leading cause of hemorrhagic stroke is having consistently high blood pressure.

Other factors can make your blood pressure worse when you have diabetes. People with high cholesterol have a tendency to have higher than normal blood pressure readings.

Having high cholesterol can make your blood pressure worse, which in turn increases your risk of having a stroke. That's because the bad cholesterol is known to be a factor in causing plaque to constrict blood flow within the blood vessels.

This is one reason why your doctor tells you to lower your LDL. You should raise your HDL, which is your good cholesterol, because your good cholesterol can counteract the effects of the bad cholesterol within your blood vessels.

If you're overweight, that also boosts your risk of stroke because it's linked to other factors that can cause this to happen. Your blood pressure is affected by you being overweight.

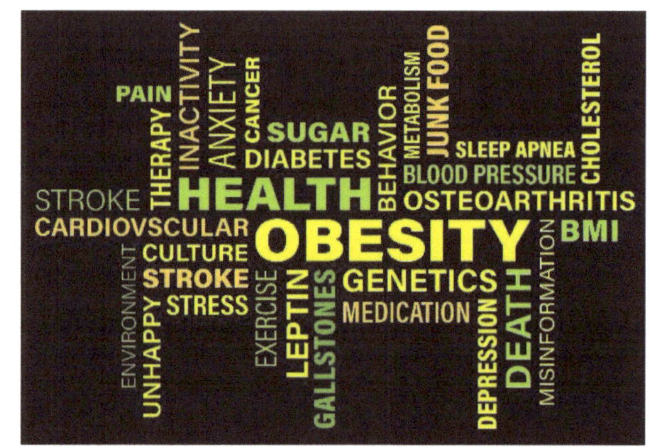

It raises your blood pressure. The more overweight you are, the harder your blood has to pump to get throughout your body. Carrying excess weight also makes your bad cholesterol rise.

There are some risks specifically associated with being overweight that can make your stroke risk factor even greater. If you're overweight, how you carry that weight on your body can determine your risk.

Men or women who are overweight and have big abdomens known as the "spare tire" or a "beer belly" are more likely to have a stroke. If your abdomen is what's known as apple shape, that also raises your risk.

Having any kind of belly fat is dangerous for diabetics, especially if you're obese. Diabetes is a disease that's linked to strokes and certain habits increase those risks. One of these habits is smoking.

This habit causes blood clots, and constricted blood flow because it can harden your blood vessels. For someone who has diabetes, there are two kinds of stroke they're most often at risk for.

One is hemorrhagic stroke and the other one is called a transient ischemic attack. This is sometimes referred to as a ministroke or TIA. Some people might blow off a TIA as no big deal since the effects of this type of stroke is not as damaging as a hemorrhagic one.

However, a TIA is simply a first step heralding the impending arrival of a stroke and should be treated just as seriously as a major stroke. The signs for either one are the same - having numbness in one arm or leg or feeling like the side of your face is numb or tingling.

Lightheadedness, dizziness and trouble maintaining your balance while walking can be a sign. Cognitive problems such as suddenly losing the ability to think clearly, communicate or understand when someone else is speaking are also telltale signs.

Some people who have a stroke will experience vision problems or get a debilitating headache. You can lower your risk of having a stroke by losing weight, getting your BMI below 30, controlling your glucose and blood pressure, eating healthy and exercising. Giving up smoking can also significantly lower your risk of a stroke.

Increased Risks of Serious Infections

Serious infections are more common in diabetics. The reason for this is because when you have diabetes, your body's immune system is compromised, so it doesn't fight back as effectively.

Not only can it not fight back as well, but the warning signs that you have an infection can be masked when you have diabetes. So you can have an infection start and you may not recognize it until you've already had it for awhile.

Common Infections for Diabetics

It's common for diabetics to get urinary tract infections (UTI). One of the reasons you may be more prone to this is because of inconsistent or high glucose levels. But you can also get a UTI if you don't completely empty your bladder when you go to the bathroom – a common problem that affects diabetics and results in the bladder breeding unhealthy bacteria.

When that happens, it can lead to another common, but more serious infection known as a bladder infection. You can tell that you have a bladder infection when you go to urinate, and the urine feels hot or you get a burning sensation.

There might also be an odor. Sometimes, when you have a yeast infection, then you can end up with a fungal bladder infection. UTIs and bladder infections might not seem like such a serious condition, but they are for diabetics.

For someone with diabetes, if these aren't treated promptly, it can lead to sepsis. Diabetics often get kidney infections. This can begin with a bladder infection and move to your kidneys.

The bacteria that causes the bladder infection is what can cause the kidney infection. Sometimes, a bladder infection can immediately turn into a kidney infection, which is then more serious.

The symptoms of a kidney infection can be mild, or they can be severe. You might have back pain, a fever or feel like you need to vomit. If the infection isn't serious, you'll be prescribed medication - but if it is serious, more aggressive treatment methods are needed.

If you have diabetes, you're more likely to develop serious infections with your feet. There are two reasons this can happen. One is because when you have diabetes, you can develop neuropathy, which includes numbness in your limbs, so you won't always feel it whenever there's a problem with your feet.

You can get hurt and have an infection start and you won't even notice it at first. The second reason is because when you have diabetes, the blood flow to the feet can become restricted, which can lead to poor circulation and swelling.

If you notice that your feet are always cold or you don't have any hair on the lower part of your legs, that's a sign. You can develop fungal infections on your feet that don't go away and these infections can spread to other parts of your body.

People who have diabetes are prone to serious skin infections as well. You can get fungal infections that can crop up between your fingers or toes. But you can also get it on or under the nails on your hands and feet.

One of the more serious skin infections is called cellulitis. This type of infection goes beyond just the surface of the skin. It goes deep into the tissues. The symptoms of cellulitis include swelling in the area and skin that looks red and is warm or hot to the touch.

You may or may not develop a fever with this condition. Cellulitis is extremely dangerous and can cause gangrene, amputation and can be fatal. People with diabetes are also more prone to severe ear and sinus infections.

Another skin infection common to diabetics is Scleroderma diabeticoru. This thickens the skin on your upper back or behind the neck. The condition Vitiligo, which discolors the skin, can also be a problem.

If you have darkened or thickened skin in some areas, such as the folds of your body, and it feels smooth and velvet-like, then you may be suffering from Acanthosis nigricans.

Many diabetics suffer from slow healing wounds, which tend to heal more quickly when your numbers are under control. Most often, it will be a foot ulcer that leads to an amputation of the foot because a simple sore becomes infected and painful.

Some of the signs that your body is fighting an infection include rashes, fevers, sores that weep, a cough that won't go away, sinus drainage, itching in the genital area or cloudy urine.

You Can Prevent Serious Infections

Having diabetes does impact your health, but you can fight back. When you're in control, you're less likely to have complications such as coming down with a serious infection.

You must understand your risks. For example, the higher your glucose levels are, the more at risk you are of getting something your body can't fight off. By keeping your sugar levels as normal as possible, you protect your immune system from damage.

That enables your body to fight off infections before they become serious. If you don't keep your levels within a healthy range, you prevent your body from fighting for you - and that includes bacterial or viral infections.

When your immune system isn't hampered by high glucose levels, it's able to keep your white blood cells healthy in order to fight foreign invaders. Besides keeping your glucose level in check, try to live as healthy a lifestyle as you possibly can.

This means you need to get and keep your weight under control. Get the exercise and sleep that you need, too. It also means that you need to watch how many carbs you eat - not only throughout the day, but at any single meal or snack time.

The carbs in a food are what hike your blood sugar levels and if you consume too many carbs, your glucose level can stay high for longer periods. Stay up to date with your shots.

Vaccines can help a diabetic fight off serious infections, such as tetanus. Those with diabetes are high risk for tetanus without the vaccine because the compromised immune system has trouble fighting off this and other bacterial infections.

Diabetics should always get the pneumonia vaccine to protect them against getting bacterial pneumonia. Certain flu vaccines can also prevent you from getting certain strains of the flu that are particularly bad for diabetics.

The Ability of Your Kidneys and Pancreas Fail to Function Properly

The kidneys are organs in the body responsible for keeping your blood clean. Much like a filter in a pool, they work to rid your body of the unhealthy things that shouldn't remain there.

But what can happen if you have diabetes is the filter process no longer works the way it should. Your kidneys can reach the point that they're no longer able to keep the waste material out of your bloodstream. When that happens, you can develop chronic problems that require dialysis and eventually, the kidneys may fail.

What Happens When Diabetes Damages Your Kidneys

There are different ways the disease can cause damage to these organs. Your kidneys have capillaries that work to keep the blood clean. It does this by preventing good by-products of your food from getting filtered out but booting out waste.

What happens over time is diabetes causes harm to these capillaries. It does this by pushing too much blood through at once. This causes the capillaries to kick into high gear and must work overtime trying to filter all that excess blood and waste.

Finally, these little gatekeepers reach the point where they start to lag, so the good by products - such as protein - escape out into your urine. This is known as proteinuria and is a warning sign for diabetics, signaling that something isn't right.

At this point, your kidneys are faltering. The blood circulating in your body is no longer being cleaned the way it should be. As a result, everything is beginning to build up. Your body is holding onto waste.

Besides causing damage to the capillaries, living with diabetes can also lead to bladder problems. The reason that you may end up with bladder problems is due to the nerves becoming damaged.

When the nerves affect your bladder, it can affect your ability to urinate. You may find that you're not able to urinate completely and the urine left in the bladder can then breed bacteria that can lead to a kidney infection.

There are symptoms that your body will give off that can alert you to the fact that something is going on with your kidneys. You might notice that when you urinate, your urine looks frothy or has a lot of bubbles in it.

If it's this way consistently, that's a sign that you're spilling a lot of protein. When your kidneys are damaged, it can make your blood pressure rise. One of the reasons for this is because of the fluid retention that occurs.

This fluid retention also causes your lower legs to ache, feeling as if they didn't rest when you went to sleep. Your legs can also swell. If you get swelling in both your ankles, that's also a symptom.

Women may experience some of the same symptoms of pregnancy - such as getting morning sickness. They may feel nauseated when they wake up or at various times throughout the day.

If you develop anemia, that's a sign of kidney problems. Experiencing unexplained itching, especially on the lower legs, is a common sign that your kidneys are no longer working right.

The itching is caused by the waste building up. Your kidneys aren't the only organs that can lose their ability to function properly. Diabetes can also cause your pancreas to have limited function.

Diabetes and Your Pancreas

The job of the pancreas is to make insulin. Without the right amount of insulin, you can develop trouble regulating your blood glucose, which is what eventually leads to diabetes.

Your body's metabolic process works by prodding the pancreas to make insulin. These beta cells get to work to take the glucose that's in your body and use it as fuel for your muscles.

It also breaks down the glucose for use in your organs. When the pancreas is affected by diabetes, it disrupts the process or work that the beta cells are supposed to do. Diabetes results in a process in which the pancreas is called on to produce more and more insulin because it's trying to combat rising blood sugar levels.

In people with diabetes, the glucose remains in the bloodstream rather than reaching the muscles and organs. The reason this happens is pretty simple. The pancreas keeps trying to get the beta cells to cover the higher glucose levels with insulin, but diabetes causes the body to resist the process.

This is why you'll hear the term insulin resistance. The higher the blood glucose levels, the harder the pancreas works trying to keep up. This causes the beta cells to start to burn out.

The more beta cells that are lost, the higher the glucose level will go. So it's a cycle of not enough insulin, the push for more, and damaging the cells, which deepens the amount of insulin that's lacking.

Eventually, this over prodding by the body for the pancreas to give it more insulin ends with the pancreas unable to do much of anything. At this point, insulin is prescribed. This process isn't something that happens overnight.

It takes years for the pancreas to reach the point where it's incapable of keeping up with the demand for glucose. What you must keep in mind is that the level at which your pancreas will function depends on whether or not your diabetes is controlled.

People who constantly have high glucose levels end up with fewer beta cells in the pancreas than people who practice good diabetes management. By sticking with a diabetic care routine, you can minimize the impact diabetes has on your pancreas.

Nerve Damage Risk Increases With Type 2 Diabetes

Your nerves can be damaged by diabetes. When that happens, the condition is referred to as diabetic neuropathy. When it comes to this side effect of living with diabetes, many people assume that it has to do with the nerves in the extremities - that they'll feel pain in their arms, hands, legs and feet.

But that's not the end of nerve damage that happens when you're a diabetic. You need to be educated about what all this entails so you can watch for signs and symptoms that your disease is out of control.

The True Effects of Nerve Damage

The problem with your diabetes reaching the stage where nerve damage occurs is that it can go inward. You can end up having nerve problems with your organs. Diabetic neuropathy can affect your entire gastrointestinal system.

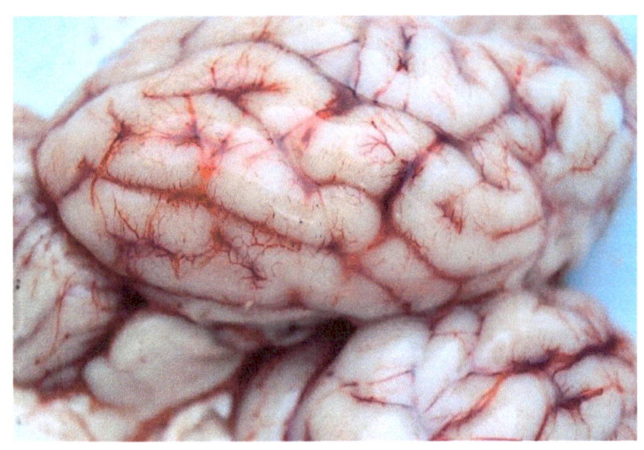

It can interfere with your body's ability to send or receive messages that relay and start or stop certain functions. For example, in your digestive tract, diabetes can cause you to end up with chronic constipation.

The nerves that function within your system can get damaged. Then your digestive tract doesn't get the signals it should. Besides constipation, diabetic neuropathy can cause diarrhea.

That's because nerve damage can get in the way of the signals that control the way your body digests foods. You can develop gastroparesis - known as a slow emptying of the stomach - if you have neuropathy.

This can make you feel full, even when it's been hours since you last ate. That's because the food in your stomach isn't moving along like it's supposed to. This can have an impact on your glucose levels.

This type of nerve damage is known as autonomic neuropathy and the biggest factor for developing this is having diabetes. While the nerve damage can cause problems with your digestive system, it can also impact your heart.

It can cause your heart rate to become abnormal. You may experience high heart rates known as tachycardia or low heart rates known as bradycardia. The disease can also damage your blood vessels because of the neuropathy.

Your bladder can be impacted, too. The nerves that are supposed to relay signals to your bladder can stop working right when they're damaged. As a result of this, it can cause the muscles that are supposed to keep urine where it belongs to function poorly.

When this happens, you'll develop incontinence. Many people who live with diabetes don't realize that the disease can also cause trouble in their sex life. Diabetes can disrupt the function of the nerves that are responsible for sexual health.

Women with the disease can experience incontinence during intimacy. They can also have little or no sex drive. Dryness can be a problem and inability to have an orgasm can also be caused by diabetic neuropathy.

Men with diabetic nerve damage can have trouble with impotence, testosterone levels, and retrograde ejaculation. The area where the nerve damage is located within your body will determine the extent of problems that you'll have as a result.

There are several warning signs that can notify someone with diabetes that there's a problem going on with the nerves. One of the symptoms of nerve damage is numbness in your hands, fingers or feet.

You can also feel numbness in your lips. You may have a sensation like you're burning under your skin. Neuropathy can also cause pain in the muscles or muscle weakness. You may feel dizzy or like you're tilting as you walk.

But you might also experience dizziness when you stand up. Nerve damage can cause bloating or a lack of hunger. You can also have problems either sweating too profusely or not sweating enough when you need to. Back pain is common with diabetic neuropathy and so is pain in the abdominal area.

Causes of and Prevention of Nerve Damage

Sometimes, diabetes is looked at with a fatalistic viewpoint - that if you have disease, the writing is on the wall. There's a false belief is that you're 100% for sure going to have the well-known complications the disease is famous for.

But your risk factors for getting neuropathy or having it worsen are under your control. You can't fix what you're not aware of. So if you had nerve damage before you were diagnosed, there's not a lot that you can do about that.

However, if you have some damage already, it doesn't have to progress. You can stop it from spreading to other parts of your body and affecting more of your organs. Your risk factor jumps considerably when you don't have a diabetic treatment plan.

It's a disease that doesn't have to get the best of you, but it will if you don't aggressively fight back. That means that you must properly maintain your glucose levels. High numbers are the top thing that can lead to nerve damage that escalates as the years pass.

The higher your numbers, the more damage you'll experience. But you don't have to live that way. Diabetes itself won't damage your body or shorten your life. Not taking care of yourself while having the disease is what will.

Check your BMI. If it's higher than normal, get it down to a normal range for your weight and height. It's true that diabetes has the ability to damage your nerves. It's also true that it can happen without outward symptoms for years.

The damage can be going on silently and you might not even know it. But that's why you should keep track of your glucose readings using your monitor. If you notice more readings that are in high ranges, that's a sign that your nerve damage risk is elevated. By taking charge, you can end the damage before it's too bad.

Ensuing Vision Problems with Type 2 Diabetes

When you have diabetes, your risk for developing vision problems is high. You can have things occur such as eye infections that can impact your ability to see. But you're also at risk for more serious problems.

You can develop eye conditions that can cause damages to your eyes. This is one reason why your doctor as well as diabetes organizations recommend seeing your ophthalmologist for an in-depth eye exam on a regular basis.

That includes right upon your diagnosis so that he or she can track changes in your vision over time. Many problems, if caught early enough, can have much less of an impact on your vision.

Some people with diabetes think that vision problems are something that happens to elderly people who have the condition. But you can develop vision related problems caused by diabetes as early as in your 20s.

There are some vision problems caused by diabetes that are temporary and easy to fix. They *are* a warning sign, however, that your glucose levels are not being controlled. If you've noticed that your vision is blurry, it can be easy to assume that your vision has simply changed if you wear corrective contact lenses or glasses.

But blurry vision is a sign that your glucose levels need immediate attention. If you notice that you've been having blurry vision, you need to go get checked to rule out any other eye problems other than elevated glucose.

Glaucoma is common in people who have diabetes. One of the reasons that's behind the development of this condition is high eye pressure. It's caused because the fluid in your eye is putting pressure on the nerves.

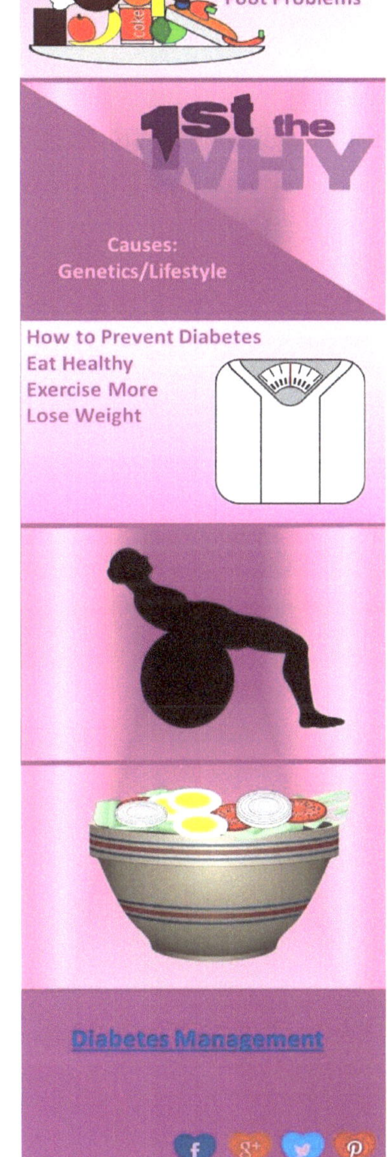

There are some well-known symptoms of glaucoma. These include pain or a feeling of pressure behind one or both eyes. You can have higher pressure in one eye than in the other.

Your vision may be blurry. This can be a result of diabetes damaging the nerves in the eye. You may also notice that your eyes are watering frequently. Losing some of your vision is also common.

The high eye pressure caused by glaucoma is treatable with medication. If you get treated, then the symptoms will go away. But you will always have to watch your eye pressure if you have this.

Left untreated, glaucoma does cause blindness. Another vision problem that results from diabetes is cataracts. You might think that having cataracts is a condition that's more common in older people, but those who have diabetes are more likely to develop cataracts earlier in life.

A cataract dims your vision. You may notice that colors aren't as bright. When you try to read print material, you may notice that the font isn't as dark when you look at it straight on.

The condition causes blurry vision. It can also cause problems with glare so that you lose the ability to do things like drive at night. Night vision impairment is one of the symptoms of the condition.

Cataracts can develop slowly over the years, but when people with diabetes get cataracts, the process is faster. You can lose your vision within a matter of several months versus over the years.

The treatment for cataracts is a short, simple eye surgery in which the surgeon will remove your cataract and you'll be given a new eye lens. Besides high glucose levels being one of the culprits that can cause vision problems, you can also develop damage simply from living with diabetes as you age.

One type of damage often labeled retina damage, is called diabetic retinopathy and it can lead to vision problems. The condition is common for diabetics. It's caused by glucose levels that are too high, injuring the blood vessels.

Problems with your retina can have more than one cause. If your blood vessels, but not your vision, are impacted by your diabetes then you still have the chance to protect your sight.

You can develop an injury caused by diabetes to the macula part of your eye. If this happens, it causes vision problems. Diabetes is also known to cause retinal detachment.

When the condition first begins to develop, you might not have any symptoms or warning signs at all. Or you might pass off the ones that you do have as no a big deal. One of the first signs is the development of floaters.

You can start to get floaters even as a child, so many people don't fret when they notice these in the eye or eyes. But with diabetes, what happens is that the floaters get worse as the foundation for retinal detachment begins.

From there, you might start to notice that your visual field appears distorted. What you look at just doesn't look normal. You can also have wavy or blurry vision. This condition also causes aneurysms in the eye.

Because these aneurysms happen where you can't see them, you might not be aware at first. As they occur, the blood vessels in the eye start to develop small circle areas that look like little balloons.

If the balloon bursts, it can lead to bleeding in the retina. This condition, if not treated right away, does cause blindness that often can't be reversed. If you have a retinal detachment, you need emergency care.

While you will not regain the vision that you lost, you can stop more vision loss from happening. If you have good diabetes management, and you make sure you have your eyes checked regularly, your chances of developing diabetic retina damage or other eye damage is less of a risk.

For people who do have diabetes, keeping your glucose levels under control, maintaining a healthy weight and having an active lifestyle can also minimize the risk. Warning signs that tell you that you need to seek the help of an eye doctor include symptoms such as a sudden infusion of multiple floaters, a burst of light like fireworks going off, consistent eye pain and any sudden changes in your visual acuity.

Skin Issues as a Diabetic

Your skin is your body's largest organ. The purpose of your skin is to keep you safe. The construction of your skin has three parts. The top is known as your epidermis. The next layer is the dermis - and finally, you have the fat section that makes up your inner skin.

When it's healthy, your skin does a good job of preventing toxins on the outside of your body from making their way inside your body and possibly making you sick or injuring you.

Without your skin, you would quickly succumb to whatever wanted to invade your body. Besides toxin protection, your body's skin works to keep you safe from the sun. It also cools you off in the summer and warms you in the winter.

This organ acts as a message center alerting your body to pain, or to temperature changes. When your skin is cared for and healthy, it's your first line of defense. Your skin is an immune system aid.

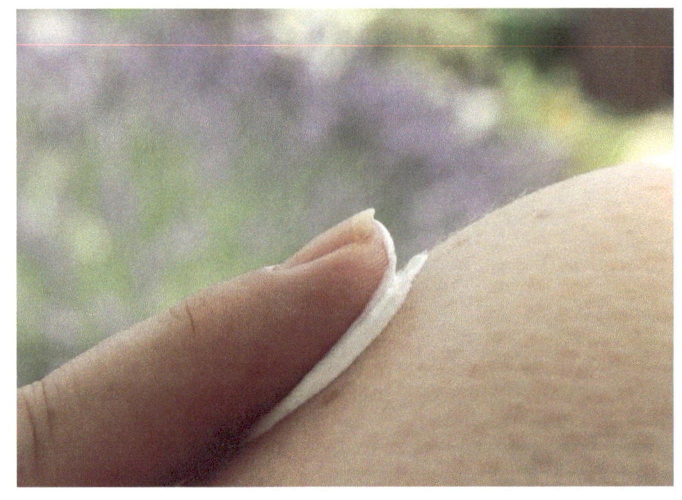

It stands guard for you against bacteria that would try to sneak into your body. But it also helps keep moisture within your body. If you're being squished against something, your skin delivers a message that it's being compressed and alerts you in order to protect your organs from harmful pressure.

Your skin is fluidly active, stretching as you bend or walk, stand or sit. When you have diabetes, your skin can't do the job it would normally do correctly. In fact, the skin is often the first noticeable symptom of diabetes.

You might notice that cuts or wounds on the skin just aren't healing the way that they used to. Diabetes causes problems for the skin because it can dry it out. The higher your blood sugar levels, the more issues you'll have with dry skin.

This happens because diabetes pulls the hydration out of your skin. As a result, it becomes dry. If your skin becomes too dry from diabetes, it will start to crack. At this point, your skin is no longer forming an effective barrier against outside threats.

You're then at risk for bacterial infections - including some serious ones. These infections can start at one place on the body and quickly move to other areas. The pigmentation of your skin can change as a result of diabetes and this can impair your skin's ability to protect you from the sun's ultraviolet rays.

Diabetes can cause you to develop patches of discoloration on your skin and these can vary in color. You might first dismiss these as just a collection of bumps or a spot. But these patches which are a direct result of diabetes can turn soft skin hard.

It can also make your skin painful to the touch. You may notice that your skin itches a lot when you have these patches. Because of these patches, your skin is then more susceptible to wounds as well as sun damage.

Skin that doesn't retain its correct thickness is also a problem that diabetes causes. It can lead to the skin on your body thickening more than it should. It can feel like you have extra layers of skin in certain areas.

Some people with diabetes compare the difficulty of dealing with this part of diabetes to having sandpaper patches on their body. As a result of that thickening, the skin will tighten and can restrict your movements.

This thickened skin can make the nerve endings less sensitive to pain or pressure points. Many people with diabetes first develop this condition on their hands and then slowly lose the ability to use their fingers the way that they once did.

The worst thing about this side effect of diabetes on the skin is that the thickening doesn't just stop with your hands. It can progress. When the skin begins to thicken on your arms, you can have difficulty moving them.

In some cases, the condition can appear on the torso and the face as well. If it becomes too severe, you can lose your mobility in some limbs. When it's healthy, your skin is smooth and trouble free, but diabetes can make problems appear without warning.

These problems can be things like sudden lesions or blistered skin. Even if you haven't done anything that would warrant the blistered skin, it can still occur. These blisters can spontaneously show up as a cluster or you may have them as single blisters.

You may not even be aware when these first develop. The reason for that is because of the diabetes, your skin won't give the signal that there's a blister. You won't feel them. You'll just notice them if you see them.

Some of these blisters can be small in size but others can be quite large. Diabetics who have developed neuropathy are more likely to experience these blisters than diabetics who haven't.

If you do notice that you have one, the blister and the area will need to be treated so that it doesn't lead to more complications. These blisters are always a sign that you have poor diabetes management.

Your skin can't protect you as well when you have diabetes because of the lack of proper blood flow to this important and largest organ. When you have diabetes, you just don't get the same amount of blood flow that you used to get.

So as a result of this, you can develop skin that can becomes scaly with random patches of red, or purplish bumps. These bumps may or may not itch and scratching them can cause them to spread.

It's true that if you have diabetes, your skin is going to be under attack from the disease. But you can prevent some of the more serious issues by keeping the right blood glucose level. When you take care of your diabetes, your skin is then able to take care of you.

Changes to the Reproductive Systems as a Diabetic

A woman's normal reproductive system can be hindered from working correctly and severely damaged by diabetes. When a woman's reproductive system is working properly, healthy egg cells are produced.

If the woman chooses not to conceive at the time, then a normal menstruation cycle occurs and the process will begin again the following month. If the woman chose pregnancy, when the egg cells are produced, they're then fertilized within the fallopian tubes.

Once fertilization is complete, if all is well, the egg travels to the uterus and is attached. These steps depend on how healthy the system is. When the egg is viable and the system is healthy, then the end result will be a pregnancy.

If the reproductive system is impacted by diabetes, it can be hindered from working correctly. If enough damage from diabetes has been done, it can make everything from having a regular or normal menstrual cycle to ovulating to conception difficult or even improbable.

Some women have conditions as a direct result of diabetes that can completely stop their monthly cycle, so the reproductive system's processes are interrupted. One of the many interruptions that can happen with the reproductive system when you have diabetes is that the disease can directly affect the hormones.

These hormones can also impact your glucose levels, so it can become a cycle that interrupts every reproductive process that's supposed to occur. For example, the disease can affect the glucose that then affects testosterone in both men and women.

When a woman has low testosterone as a result of diabetes, not only will she lack sex drive, but she'll also have trouble with other hormones associated with reproduction. A man's reproductive hormones are also affected by diabetes.

When that happens, men will experience some of the symptoms of menopause when they have diabetes associated damage to their reproductive system. They can experience flashes of heat and can have the sweats.

They may also have fatigue or a lack of interest in intimacy. They may also experience mood swings as if they were experiencing a monthly cycle. The loss of testosterone can cause their breast tissue to grow and they can end up developing breasts.

They may also experience other signs of reproductive system damage such as gaining fat in the midsection. Men who have diabetes, especially if the glucose levels aren't controlled, can face some or all of that list of reproductive problems.

However, one of the main issues that affects men with diabetes is erectile dysfunction. That's because the disease can cause damage to the nerves or blood flow in the male reproductive system.

This can lead to weakness with erections. When they experience problems maintaining an erection, most men don't realize that this can be a sign of uncontrolled diabetes. They're also unaware that if they practice good diabetes management, the problem will resolve when the blood sugars are normalized.

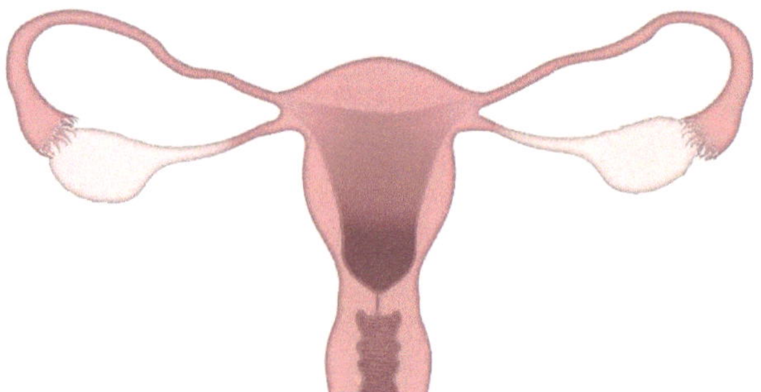

Sometimes, if it's extensive, the damage that's already been done due to the diabetes cannot be reversed - but the good news is that getting the disease under control can stop the condition from getting worse.

Diabetes can also cause other health issues in the reproductive organs of both men and women, which can sometimes greatly impact fertility. For women, one of the issues that diabetes is linked to is problems with the ovaries.

Without good ovarian health, it can wreak havoc on a women's entire reproductive system. It can cause erratic or zero ovulation. Diabetes can lead to high androgen levels and it also cause arrested development of follicles.

This then causes the eggs that are released to be inferior. That's followed by a further inability to conceive. Most women who have diabetes understand that if their disease is not well controlled, it can result in reproductive system problems - including limiting their chances of getting pregnant.

But what they and their partner may not realize is that diabetes can also damage the DNA in sperm, which can cause difficulty with conception. Many couples are unaware that high levels of glucose could be the root cause of the fertility issues they may be experiencing.

There's a reason that diabetes affects male fertility. In a reproductive study, high glucose levels were shown to be the cause of damage within a man's sperm DNA. This damage raises infertility odds.

In a healthy man, the body would naturally work to repair any DNA that's damaged. But the body's ability to repair its DNA is weakened when someone has diabetes. Because of this, the sperm cannot be made viable again.

So men who have uncontrolled diabetes can then be infertile. The study also showed that when the DNA is damaged by diabetes, if a pregnancy does somehow occur, there's another risk.

This risk is a higher than normal chance of having a miscarriage. The study also showed that when men or women are obese, the diabetes can affect the ability of the sperm to reach the egg for fertilization.

Diabetes can also affect sperm density and the lower a man's count, the greater the difficulty in conceiving. Diabetes doesn't have to cause problems with the reproductive system and it doesn't have to cause fertility issues. But unless it's managed correctly, it will do just that and worse.

Increased Risk of Dental Issues When Living with Diabetes

Diabetes isn't a disease that's simply about your body's inability to function properly with the insulin your pancreas does or doesn't produce. It's not a disease that's the same for every person.

Some might take oral medications, and some might need to take insulin. But one thing is true regardless of where you are with your diabetes - even if you're the most careful person in the world with monitoring your diabetes, you can still have dental problems.

The Effects of Diabetes on Your Mouth

When you have diabetes, you're more likely to have problems with dental issues because your body can't fight back the way it could if you didn't have the disease. So as a result of that, you'll find that you may have issues that affect your oral health.

The more uncontrolled your diabetes is, the worse your dental issues will be. A well known side effect of living with diabetes is dry mouth. This is known as xerostomia and you can have it regardless of the age you are, how long you've had diabetes or the type of diabetes that you have.

There are several signs that you might not be aware of that signal you have dry mouth. One of these symptoms is trouble swallowing food. This happens because the condition of dry mouth can present itself as a lack of saliva.

Since saliva is needed to break down the food that you eat, not having enough can make it difficult to chew and swallow your food. Saliva is also needed to help prevent cavities.

When you don't have enough saliva, you're more prone to developing both plaque and cavities. With dry mouth, you may notice that your tongue looks different. It can take a dry, cracked appearance and you may notice this same result with your lips.

It's also common for diabetes to affect your mouth by causing painful sores or infections. You can develop gingivitis or painful gums. This is caused because having diabetes means that your body has a weakened immune system and isn't able to fight off the inflammation or bacteria that commonly affect the teeth and gums.

As a diabetic, you're at a higher risk of developing periodontal disease. This infection is deep below the surface and can cause serious damage not only to your gums but to your bones as well.

If it's not caught and treated early, the disease can cause your jawbones to become weak. Having periodontal disease can also make your glucose levels rise. The good news is that this and other mouth issues can be treated and controlled if you keep your sugar levels in a healthy range.

You should also stay away from things that can worsen mouth issues - such as drinking caffeine or alcohol. You should also make sure that you're drinking plenty of liquid. Not getting at least 8 glasses of water daily can exacerbate mouth problems.

Any time you have a spot in your mouth that doesn't heal quickly, you should always have your dentist check it out. Because of your diabetes, it can be easier to get a serious mouth infection.

What You Can Do to Fight Back Against Dental Issues

When you have diabetes, you always have to be on the offensive with your health - and that includes your dental health. You want to practice good habits and take care of any problems as soon as you become aware of them.

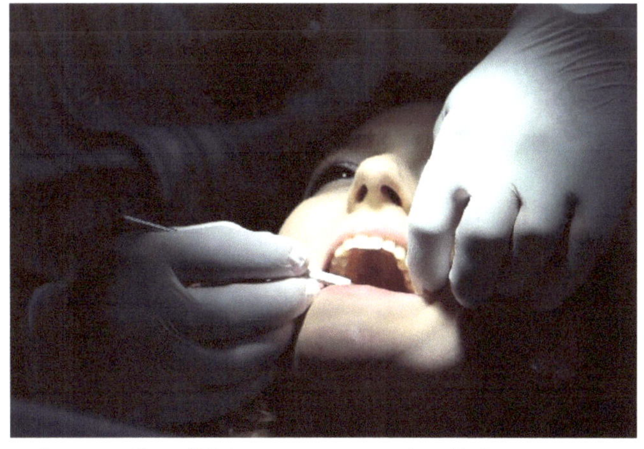

That means you have to make sure that you keep up with your regular dental appointments. It's important for diabetics to get their teeth checked every six months. This way, your dentist can spot any problems before they become big issues.

Besides practicing good day to day control over your blood sugar levels, you need to know what your A1C levels are. This test shows an average of what your ranges were for the prior three months.

By having this test, you can determine if you're practicing good glucose control. If it's too high, then these results can often alert you to a problem with your dental health long before you even know you have one.

Once you have the results, you can talk to your dentist about them and greater care can be taken to check for underlying and often hidden health problems with your gums. One way to fight back against dental issues starts by watching what you eat.

You don't have to give up your favorite foods, but you need to eat healthy and this means watching the amount of carbs that you eat every day. Eating a diet that helps control your glucose levels allows you to fight back against any potential dental issues.

When your levels are under control, your body is better able to fight the bacteria and infections in the mouth so you won't be as prone to having dental problems. Make exercise a habit because this can help your body use the glucose rather than it staying in the bloodstream.

Give up any habits that can worsen dental issues. These would be habits like smoking, which makes a diabetic more vulnerable to poor dental health. Smoking causes problems with the blood flow in the mouth.

Give up habits that bathe your teeth constantly in sugar, such as chewing gum made with sugar or keeping hard candies in your mouth for prolonged periods of time. If you use a hard toothbrush, give it up and instead, brush your teeth with a soft toothbrush.

People who have diabetes are prone to gum problems and brushing with a hard toothbrush can cause a gum irritation. Due to the diabetes, that irritation is more likely to turn into an infection. As a diabetic, it's better to floss after every meal but at least floss twice a day if you can't.

The Emotional Well-Being at Risk

Discovering that you have diabetes can throw your emotions into a tailspin. The disease itself - plus dealing with it - can feel like such a heavy burden that it can put your emotional well-being at risk.

Emotions Linked to Diabetes

Type 2 diabetes can send many people into a state of grief - both those who are newly diagnosed as well as people who've lived with the condition for years. When you discover that you have it, you'll go through the stages of grieving the life that you once had and this is a normal reaction.

But if you've had the disease for awhile, you can reach the point where you just get tired of the disease and you can start to grieve everything that's now different and everything you've had to put up with.

One emotion linked to diabetes is denial. This can happen in both the early stage of discovery as well as striking out of the blue after having dealt with it for months or years. People just decide that they don't want the disease, so they convince themselves that they don't have it or that everything will be fine.

Another emotion linked to diabetes is anger. People who have diabetes can sometimes feel angry at having the disease and all the side effects that go hand in hand with the condition.

They might get annoyed seeing someone else who is overweight who doesn't have the disease and wonder why they didn't so lucky. This anger can impact a person physically.

When you get angry, it can raise your glucose levels. It can make your heart pound and anger that isn't treated can lead to a heart attack if you're under enough emotional duress.

Anger can cause you to have headaches, problems with sleeping and eating, it can also lead to anxiety and depression. Diabetes can cause anxiety. The anxiety can raise your glucose levels and lead to problems keeping it under control.

It can cause you to feel worried about managing the disease, which leads to greater anxiety and high glucose levels. It's common to struggle with depression when you have diabetes.

The more out of control your glucose numbers are, the more you can suffer from depression. It acts like a catch-22. When you feel depressed, you don't want to deal with your diabetes and when you don't deal with your diabetes, you feel depressed.

You also feel worse physically as the higher numbers take a toll on your body. Whatever emotions that diabetes is causing in your life, you have to deal with it - otherwise, your health will worsen.

You can start to have fatigue and trouble concentrating. Your weight can fluctuate, and both weight gain and weight loss can impact your diabetes. You may lose interest in food or find that you're overeating and just don't care.

Diabetes puts your emotional well-being at risk because it can cause you to feel like it's

the worst thing in the world and that nothing will ever get better. You may find that you're closing yourself off.

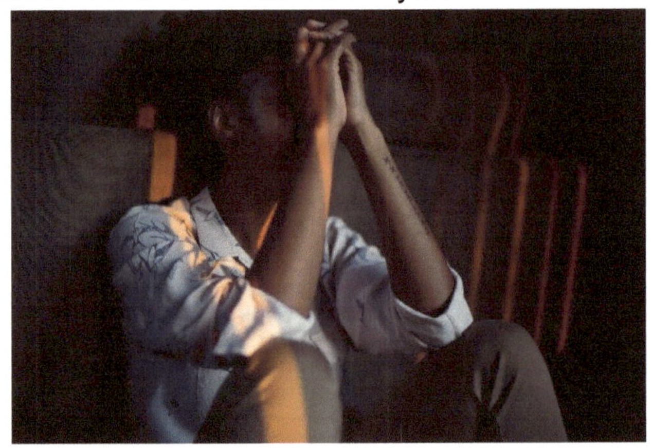

You might stop doing things that you once enjoyed doing and just stop practicing good diabetes care. Diabetes can drain you emotionally because of all the stuff you have to deal with to take care of yourself.

Why You Must Deal With Diabetes For Your Emotional Well-Being

Diabetes isn't the kind of condition that you can just blow off. You can't just sort of take care of yourself once or twice a week. It's a daily thing, taking care of your diabetes. You have to deal with your condition in order to have good emotional well-being.

There are many options that you can use to help not only come to terms with living with diabetes but taking care of yourself physically as well. You can do things like practice meditation or mindfulness.

You can take up yoga or a hobby. But whatever you do, don't just avoid dealing with whatever it is that your diabetes is causing you to feel. Because if you don't, you can get what's called diabetes burnout.

This is what happens when you reach the point where you feel you just can't take it anymore. You're tired of the constant vigilance in making sure that you take care of your diabetes.

You can feel like you're always having to watch your step. This happens because diabetes puts you under a lot of stress physically, which makes you feel stress emotionally.

And if you don't deal with it, you can reach the place in your life when you feel like throwing your hands up and declaring that you're done. This is a normal reaction, too - but you can't give up.

Instead, you must decide that you're going to find ways to deal with your diabetes that give you the best health possible. When you do that, your emotional well-being will benefit.

You can start by realizing that you're never going to achieve 100% accuracy in anything you do to take care of yourself. There will be days when you're not going to want to eat in a way that's best for your disease.

That's normal. But what you must realize is that 28 days in a month taking care of your diabetes is still better than giving up altogether. There will be times when things are going to go on with your body because of the diabetes.

As a result, you're not always going to have glucose levels that are where you want them to be. What you have to do is to accept that one high glucose reading does not make you a failure and it doesn't mean your diabetes is out of control.

What you have to learn is that taking care of your diabetes is taking care of your emotions. When you eat right, exercise, and get the right amount of sleep, you're going to feel more empowered. If you feel more empowered, your mental health will be better. If your mental health is better, than so will be your physical health as the brain controls everything that goes on in the body.

Final Thoughts

There you have it – the possible complications when faced with a Type 2 diabetes diagnosis. With that information in mind on what could happen, lets wrap up this book with some information on how to best minimize the risk of complications. As we see below, exercise is very important for diabetics.

Exercise Plan for Diabetes Control

Adopting an exercise program is important in every person's life no matter if they're disabled or have the body of an athlete. But for a diabetic, it could mean life and death. A diagnosis of diabetes means that you have to change your lifestyle to combat the risk of developing even more serious health problems.
Exercise plans that combine slow-paced exercises such as Yoga with exercises that increase cardiovascular fitness are essential to manage your diabetes properly. It's important to take steps to prevent injury in any exercise plan you choose, but even more so with diabetics since wound healing is worsened and slower than normal.

The Important Role of Exercise in Diabetes Management

Everyone should know by now that exercise is an important part of maintaining or losing weight and keeping healthy. Exercise has an even more important role for diabetics in managing your blood sugar and avoiding insulin resistance.
Many times those with type 2 diabetes are producing some insulin, but not enough for what they require. Weight loss, exercise and lifestyle changes can help make a difference in how much insulin you need. You may even be able to get the glucose levels back to normal – without extra insulin or meds.

Exercises should be performed regularly to realize the benefits. Those diabetics who exercise on a regular basis experience less risk for a stroke or heart attack. And when you exercise, your muscles are busy using sugar and oxygen – which helps insulin work as it should.

Both types of exercise – aerobic and anaerobic – make you stronger. If you haven't exercised in awhile, Yoga exercises or stretching can help you get started. Then, when you feel up to it, you can choose from aerobic or anaerobic.

Aerobic exercise causes the body to use large amounts of oxygen, lowering blood pressure, blood lipids and blood sugar that aren't needed. Some aerobic exercises include swimming, dancing, jogging or anything you can do to get your heart rate up. In anaerobic exercise, you're working one area of the body at a time in short energy bursts. You can build muscles with anaerobic exercises, but it doesn't strengthen lungs or your heart.

And you don't use enough blood sugar to make a difference in your blood sugar levels. Regular exercise, along with a healthy diet, is the best thing you can do for yourself to keep healthy and fit.

For the diabetic, it's imperative if you want to keep your blood sugar under control.

Exercise metabolizes the glucose in your body and maintains normal blood sugar level. Your body will function more effectively because it helps increase intensity of insulin to the tissue in those suffering from type 2 diabetes.

That means more glucose leaves the bloodstream and travels into cells where it's used for the purpose of creating energy. So the glucose in the blood is reduced, which is a very good thing for diabetics.

Exercise helps build muscles, which also use glucose to maintain their working order. So exercise helps the muscles gain the glucose needed and, in turn, lowers the blood sugar level.

Don't forget that exercise burns fat and calories - which help you maintain a healthy weight. When you manage to maintain a healthy weight, your blood sugar level can stay in the normal range.

You may have trouble getting started on an exercise program if you've never been in to it before. Have patience and try new things until you find a program that works for you. Then, mix it up and try some new exercises that you might enjoy.

It's Crucial to Monitor Your Blood Sugar with Exercise

Just as exercise is important to diabetics, the act of monitoring your blood sugar before and after exercise is crucial. Whether you eat before or after an exercise session can raise or lower the levels drastically.

You should definitely check your blood sugar levels before and after exercise – and also during the workout. You'll then know how your body is reacting to exercise and that will help you prevent wide and potentially dangerous swings in your blood sugar levels.

If you've been inactive for awhile, be sure and check with your doctor before jumping into any exercise activity. He can direct you about the best time to exercise and how any medications you may be taking would affect your blood sugar.

For diabetics, the recommended amount of exercise to reap the most benefits is approximately 12 ½ hours per week of such exercises as swimming, bicycling or brisk walking.

Those who are taking insulin or other medications to lower blood sugar should test blood sugar 30 minutes before exercise begins. If your blood sugar is too low (lower than 100 mg/dL) at that time, you should try eating a snack of low carbs (up to 30 grams) before beginning your exercise program.

If your blood sugar measures 100 to 250 mg. or higher, you can begin your exercise routine. When your blood sugar is too high (250 mg/dL) you should take all precautions before you can exercise. That means testing your urine for the presence of ketones, which indicate your body can't control your blood sugar for lack of insulin.

With ketones at a high level, you risk the condition of ketoacidosis, which needs immediate treatment. Ketoacidosis is a serious complication for diabetics, so be sure to attempt to get your blood sugar levels down before exercising.

During exercise, monitor your blood sugar every half hour and watch for symptoms of low blood sugar. This is true especially if you're planning to work out for a long period of time or the workout intensity increases.

Stop exercising if your blood sugar level is at a dangerous number. Soon, you'll get to know how your body responds to exercise (such as feeling weak or confused) and be able to more accurately predict what impact exercise has on your blood sugar levels.

When you finish your exercise routine, check your blood sugar immediately. Keep checking several times in the next few hours. Exercise removes sugar held in your liver and muscles and when your body restores that sugar, it must take the sugar from your blood.

Your blood sugar is more affected the longer or more strenuous your exercise is. You may have low blood sugar for up to eight hours after you finish exercising. Have a snack such as nuts or a granola bar after the workout to keep your blood sugar from fluctuating.

How Much Exercise Does a Diabetic Need?

All diabetics should exercise to get the benefits it offers in lowering your blood sugar and strengthening your body. Experts recommend that 150 minutes (about 12 hours) of mid-intensity aerobic exercise (activity that raises your heart rate) per week is a good goal to shoot for.

Whatever days you choose for exercising, you should try to schedule it for the same time and same day every week. Your body will get used to the changes in blood sugar levels and be better able to control it naturally.

If you're taking insulin, a set time and day will help you better regulate insulin intake. Some diabetics are also dealing with obesity and exercise can be very beneficial to reduce weight.

Some diabetics with type 2 diabetes have been able to successfully lose weight on a carefully monitored exercise and diet plan. Blood sugar levels can become regulated enough so there is no more need for insulin and medications.

Choose a type of exercise that's enjoyable to you and you'll have less risk of getting bored and discontinuing it. Keep in mind that diabetics should consider the stress that certain exercises have on the feet, something that poses a problem for those with this diagnosis.

A sedentary lifestyle puts everyone at risk for being overweight and subject to a great number of diseases. Exercise can help both in weight loss and works to keep diseases at bay.

Although the benefits of exercise are widely known, the diabetic should take extra precautions not to overexert or tire the body too much. Stop exercising immediately if you feel any type of discomfort in any part of your body.

Numbness, pain or annoying tingling in your legs should also be an alert for you to stop exercising. Extreme weather can also make a difference in the risk of you developing hypoglycemia. Cold weather can make the skin dry and cracked, which isn't good for a diabetic.

Any other changes in the way your body functions should also be considered during exercise. For example, if you become short of breath or nauseated, don't exercise or stop immediately. Dizziness or light-headedness and confusion are also red flags for the diabetic.

Why Walking and Weight Training Are Effective Diabetes Controllers

There are good reasons why walking and weight training are the best choices for diabetics. Exercise strengthens bodies and can control blood glucose levels. One of the best reasons is that exercise can significantly lengthen your life span.

Simply adding walking to your lifestyle can reduce your risk of death from any cause in up to 40% of diabetics if you spend two hours a week walking. Even if you just walk a couple of times a week, brisk walking can effectively help reduce blood sugar levels.

Among other great benefits, walking also improves circulation so important to diabetics and prevents fat cells from forming. Take precautions when taking up walking to choose the right type of walking shoes to prevent injury or cause blisters on the feet.

Weight training is a great muscle builder. For each pound of muscle you gain, your body will burn approximately 50 more calories even when you're not working out. That's a boon to diabetics who want to lose weight.

Muscles also help diabetics by taking glucose away from the bloodstream for their own purpose. When the muscles take the glucose, the blood sugar level is naturally lowered. Another benefit of weight training is that it increases metabolism helping you energetic and youthful.

Weight training and building muscle as a result also reduces your risk of injury by increasing your strength. Injuries are a major concern for diabetics because it takes longer for the healing process.

Walking and weight training also improve bone density, lower blood pressure, keep the gastrointestinal tract functioning properly and reduce the risk of heart disease and cancer.

Especially helpful to the diabetics, walking and weight training improves the condition of insulin resistance. A diabetic who exercises judiciously can expect to enjoy better health and a better chance of controlling blood sugar levels.

Exercises That Prevent Injury and Ensure Success for Diabetics

Exercise can be particularly tough on the diabetic because of the chance of injury or doing damage to the feet. Injuries are more difficult to heal for the diabetic, so if you're going to exercise, make sure it's a routine that has a lower risk of injury and ensures the success that exercising can bring to the body.

Swimming, the stationary bike and weight training are good choices because they get your heart rate up and build muscle. You may need specialized shoes if you choose walking to be sure you don't get blisters. And be sure to wear socks.

Those exercises not recommended for diabetics - include parachuting, diving and mountain or rock climbing. All of these types of exercises increase the chances of injury and could cause hypoglycemia, which can lead to very serious diabetic complications.

Types of aerobic exercises that get the heart rate up are good choices for diabetics. Aerobic activity helps you manage hypertension and can reduce cholesterol to lower the risk of stroke or heart disease.

A diabetic is especially subject to depression, lack of self-esteem and dementia. Exercise releases endorphins which boost mental health and confidence and lowers the risk of depression. Exercise also helps to alleviate stress.

Good, quality sleep is also important for the diabetic to be able to have the energy and peace of mind to manage the many tasks of dealing with diabetes. Always listen to your body to tell you when you shouldn't exercise.

Testing blood sugar is important to find out if it's a good time for exercise or if you should wait until the blood sugar levels out. And if you're suffering from an infection or a severe and open wound, don't exercise until the doctor tells you it's healed.

Becoming an active exerciser might mean that you have to overcome some obstacles - such as not having enough time or energy, but when you're able to overcome the barriers and get yourself on a regular exercise routine, you'll notice a big difference in the way you feel and the ease in which you can keep your blood sugar regulated.

If you're a diabetic, be sure to discuss any type of exercise you choose with a doctor before engaging in it. Exercise doesn't have to cost anything and it will have an immediate impact on your health and well-being.

Low Carb for Diabetes Control

A diagnosis of diabetes means that your body doesn't properly process the sugars in food and you need to adopt a diet plan that can also provide the body with energy and growth. The three types of diabetes include type 1, type 2 and gestational. Each requires a different medical plan of action.

A low-carb diet is considered best for most diabetics, but a complete diet plan for your diabetes condition may be totally different from another diabetic's. Be sure you do the research, discuss your condition with your doctor and develop the right plan for you.

How Carbs Impact a Diabetic's Blood Sugar

The impact of carbs on a diabetic's blood sugar is simple to understand. Your body breaks down the sugar and turns it into energy when you're not a diabetic, but when you are, is accumulates in your blood – causing high blood sugar count if you consume too many carbs.

High blood sugar can cause serious complications when you have diabetes. A low carbohydrate diet can improve your blood sugar count because your body is consuming less sugar, making it easier for the body to produce natural insulin to process blood sugars.

Evidence is strong that a low carb diet can help to control type 1 and 2 diabetes.

Even if you take insulin for your diabetes condition, it's easier to control the amount needed if you consume fewer carbohydrates.
When a person with type 1 or 2 diabetes lowers carbohydrate count, insulin absorption is reduced, which reduces the amount of insulin needed in injections. Blood sugar management is essential for diabetics to keep from having severe complications.

Diabetics are urged to pay close attention to the amount of carbs they're consuming because they can affect blood sugar levels much more rapidly than fat or protein. One way people count carbs is to split the carbs you eat and drink at each meal.

You'll know that you've consumed more carbs than needed if your blood sugar goes up. You know you've given your body more than the insulin can handle. Too few carbs will lower your blood sugar.

If the count is too low, you need to increase carbs. The trick is finding a balance. It helps if you know how to count carbs and fortunately, you can get information on the label of almost any food item.

If you need to count carbs because you use insulin several times per day or have an insulin pump, keep in mind that the type of insulin you were prescribed may impact your meal planning.

There are several ways to develop a low-carb diet plan. Generally, you'll be counting carbs you consume and attempting to lower the count by adjusting your diet. You may want to ask your health care provider about a diabetes food exchange list that you can quickly access rather than having to count carbs at each meal.

Exercise is part of the strategy to lower blood sugar count and should also be a part of your lifestyle plan to fight diabetes. Exercise and diet, when used together to combat the disease, can greatly impact the severity of symptoms and future complications.

If you're like the normal person in Western civilization you're probably consuming about 50% carbohydrates (or more) in your diet and much less fat and protein. Those who are trying to control diabetes through a low-carb diet plan may eat very few carbs per day while others consume a bit more and both are able to manage their diabetes.

That's why it's important to individualize your low-carb plan as much as possible. Trial and error usually works until you know how many carbs you'll need according to your taste, energy and blood sugar levels.

The Best Carb Count for Type II Diabetes

A wide range is used to define the best carb count for type 2 diabetes. You must first test your ability to handle carbs and then decide on the right number for you. The general range of carb consumption for diabetics is between 20 and 90.

If you're new to carb counting, there are a few things you need to know about the process. It's important for diabetics to count carbs because of how they may affect your blood sugar and the medications or insulin you're taking.

Diabetics with type 1 or 2 diabetes who are required to take insulin to balance blood sugar levels should be able to match the amount of insulin you must take with carbohydrates that you consume from eating and drinking.

Those with type 2 diabetes who are not required to take insulin can count carbs to balance the carbs consumed with blood glucose levels, weight issues and any prescriptions you may be taking.

Counting carbohydrates must be done diligently if you're going to have success in adjusting your insulin or diabetic medication to keep blood glucose levels balanced. The impact that carbs have to convert what you eat into glucose is tremendous and must be balanced.

Carbs can be found in such foods as breads, pasta and other grain-based items, fruits, root vegetables such as potatoes and yams, desserts and other types of sweets, some vegetables and most dairy products.

All sugars containing fructose, maltose, dextrose and sucrose also have high carb count. Carbohydrates are usually counted using the measurement of grams. You'll find that certain foods are all carbs while others are partially carbs, protein or fats.

The carb count is the same whether you're counting from bread, fruit or other food items. Use labels on food items, a good reference book, scale and lists of carbohydrates to gather information about carb content.

There are also computer programs that offer lots of information and guidance on counting carbs. Once you get the hang of it, carb counting is easy. There are two ways you can count carbs – basic and consistent.

In each method, you'll calculate the total carbs in a food item and then match those carbs to the number that you can safely consume. Then, it's easy to figure the portion size and medications that have an impact on the count.
If you're using the basic carb counting method, you'll be able to learn how your blood glucose levels react to certain foods. The goal of carb counting is to consume a daily carb count that is consistent in helping the blood glucose levels remain balanced.

Most individuals who are diagnosed with type 2 diabetes (non-insulin) use the basic method of counting carbs. The consistent method of carb counting is extremely important for those with type 1 diabetes (with insulin).

In type 1 diabetes, the pancreas is no longer able to produce insulin, so carb count becomes extremely important and you should check with your physician or dietitian for the best way to count carbs.

Making the Right Carb Choices for a Diabetic Diet

While diabetics do need to keep track of the carbs they eat, there are certain carbs that can help create a balanced diet plan that will work for both type 1 and type 2 diabetes.

There are two types of low-carb diets – high protein and high fat – and some people combine the two into a low carb (high protein), high fat diet. High protein diabetics should find their carbs in animal protein and tofu (if vegan or vegetarian). High fat diabetics should consume cuts of meat that are fatty and also consume other foods that are high in fat such as olive oil and avocado.

Both high protein and high fat diabetics should discuss their situation with their physician because some diets that are high in protein can cause kidney problems or make kidney issues worse. Although donuts may be out of the question for a low-carb diet, those people diagnosed with diabetes can enjoy a wide variety of foods that are delicious and good for you. The low-carb diet limits your intake of high carb foods such as sweets, breads and starchy vegetables like potatoes.

You need to remember when you begin a low carb diet plan that sugar is directly converted to glucose and can raise your blood glucose levels. But, you can reduce or replace those high-carb foods by eating small portions and filling up on healthy fats, protein and vegetables that are non-starchy.
Protein and high fiber foods are nutrients that help you digest and absorb carbs, so your blood sugar levels don't spike suddenly. Foods rich in protein and fiber include lentils and beans, but beans can be high in carbs.

Black-eyed, green and split peas also contain high fiber and also give you nutrients and vitamins such as vitamin C, K, phosphorus and folate. Berries also offer a plethora of benefits for diabetics.

Some have lower sugar content than others – such as blueberries, strawberries, blackberries and raspberries. These powerful berries also offer phytonutrients like flavonoids and others that help boost your immune system.

Sweet potatoes are a diabetic's dream food. They're digested much more slowly than their white potato cousins and won't raise your blood sugar rapidly. They also are chock full of beta-carotene, which helps your immune system function properly and aids digestion.

Plain Greek yogurt contains carbs, but they are derived from the natural sugar – lactose. And, it also contains protein and calcium to boost bone health. Greek yogurt is great for diabetics who don't exercise or have other problems.

Apples and pears contain natural sugar, but also contain fiber. Try munching on these fruits dipped in peanut or almond butter. It's best not to consume the juice from these or any other fruits because they have tons of sugar and no fiber.
Winter squash like butternut, pumpkin and acorn are packed with fiber that will help keep your blood levels balanced. And, they're also full of vitamins such as manganese, beta-carotene and vitamin C.

These low-carb choices for diabetics are also great choices for those who want to manage their weight and/or become healthier. A low-carb diet can help protect your immune system and reduce risks of other diseases such as high blood pressure and cancer.

Low Carb Desserts for a Diabetic Sweet Tooth

You don't have to be a diabetic or watching your carbs to lose weight to enjoy the delicious desserts that won't have such an impact on your blood sugar. From cookies and cakes to pies and puddings, there are great recipes that are perfect for the diabetic sweet tooth.

Diabetics may think they need to stay far away from a Fat Bomb, but some can actually be good for you. When you think of a fat bomb, something like cheeseburger and fries with a chocolate shake probably comes to mind – but that's not what this is about.

Fat bombs are typically made with high fat, low carb foods. You can make things like peanut butter fat bombs, chocolate mousse fat bombs and more – and they're generally a small dessert that packs a punch in terms of satisfying your sweet tooth and also filling you up so that you're not craving anything anymore.

Certain desserts can be turned into low-carb desserts that only have 15 carb grams or less. They contain energy rather than calories so it's easier to maintain your weight – and they're healthy for you too.

They can be made with dried fruit, oats, coconut, unsweetened chocolate, nut butters and more. They're high-fat, but low-carb and very satisfying. For example, one recipe for a diabetic fat bomb is a cookie made from oats and contains coconut oil.

Then, there are the brownies made with peanut butter and chocolate made with flour substitutes, chocolate and peanut butter. When you do have a raging sweet tooth, remember that dark chocolate, sugar-free candy and ice creams such as Halo can be consumed by diabetics without fear.

High Protein, Low Carb Meals for Diabetics

When you sit down to a meal as a diabetic, you're likely assessing the meal to figure out what you can eat. One mistake that diabetics often make is not eating enough carbs. This varies from person to person and depends on your energy level and blood sugar levels.

Quality carbs count more, too. If you only eat a dessert for your daily amount of carbs, try Greek yogurt and berries for another source. When you plan your meals, be sure to include a protein such as fish or grilled chicken.

You can then add a salad or vegetables low in carbohydrates such as green salads or broccoli. You should know how many carbs you can safely consume and if you must stay on a very low carb diet, add nuts or another high fat/low carb item.

Other diabetics may want to have a portion of legumes or a root vegetable (carrots or sweet potatoes) on their plates. A low-carb fruit would also be a good choice. Whole grains like quinoa or bulgar can be a great addition, but eliminate such foods as refined pasta or grains.

Enjoying a beverage with your meal such as unsweetened herbal or iced tea, water or even a dry red wine is okay, but avoid sweet or diet beverages (with artificial sweeteners).

It takes a lot of patience and trial and error to find foods that you like and that won't raise your blood glucose levels to dangerous heights. Protein, fiber and some healthy fat on your plate can be very satisfying and a great way to watch your weight and get healthy, too.

Be sure to check your blood sugar levels at various times after eating to see how your body is responding. Also, pay attention to your energy level and whether you're satisfied after the meal.

With a little adjustment here and there, diabetics can enjoy delicious and satisfying meals and manage blood sugar with very little effort. A low-carb diet is healthy for both diabetics and non-diabetics.

Acceptable Diabetic Foods

This list is based on a low-carb diet plan, although it is not strictly low-carbs. Carbs are allowed, but try to avoid processed carbs as much as possible. Processed carbs are prepackaged foods, cakes, cookies, most breads, pasta, etc.

Proteins:

- Fish
- Shellfish
- Lean meats
- Poultry

Fruits & Vegetables:

- You can basically eat all the leafy greens you want.
- Limit the consumption of potatoes, sweet potatoes and other root vegetables.
- Limit the consumption of corn.
- Limit fruits, but have one to two servings per day.

Tip: Banana and peanut butter are a great snack and also a good source of potassium, which is important to diabetics.

Low GI Foods: Eat in moderation

- Peas, beans, legumes
- Brown rice
- Whole grains
- Steel cut oats

Other Moderation Foods: One serving per day is acceptable

- Dairy
- Nuts & Seeds

Extremely limit or avoid:

- Corn
- Potatoes
- Pasta
- Bread
- Instant oatmeal

For more information see the ADA shopping list. Please note, it has more carbohydrate foods than we've suggested here.

http://main.diabetes.org/dorg//PDFs/WeightLoss/shopping-list.pdf

Resources

As you red through the book you no doubt saw words underlined and highlighted in blue. These are links to other sources of information that you can read. Some are blog posts from my website Diabetes Management; some is free information on my website that you can download; still others are books that you can buy that I have published on diabetes and related topics either on my website or on Amazon.

The links with letters are in the Kindle ebook format, while the ones with all numbers are paperbacks such as you are reading here.

Introduction

- Diabetes Management: https://healthylifestylenewsletter.com/diabetes/
- information store: https://healthylifestylenewsletter.com/diabetes/shop/
- worsen: https://www.amazon.com/gp/product/1541232186
- lack of sleep: https://www.amazon.com/gp/product/B07KWL8F9C
- major problems: https://www.amazon.com/gp/product/1983312193/
- manage the condition: https://healthylifestylenewsletter.com/diabetes/product/managing-type-2-diabetes-using-alternative-and-natural-therapies/

Type 2 Diabetes and Your Heart

- manageable: https://healthylifestylenewsletter.com/diabetes/
- exercise: https://www.amazon.com/gp/product/1520521405
- heart: https://www.amazon.com/gp/product/B00WRCHCRS
- lose weight: https://www.amazon.com/gp/product/1718645724
- poor lifestyle choices: https://www.amazon.com/gp/product/B072L5DMCR
- Mediterranean Diet: https://www.amazon.com/gp/product/1534683119

Diabetics Have an Increased Risk of Stroke

- side effects of living with diabetes:

https://healthylifestylenewsletter.com/diabetes/scared-straight-the-most-horrific-consequences-of-obesity/

Increased Risks of Serious Infections

- neuropathy: https://www.amazon.com/gp/product/1983312193
- feet: https://healthylifestylenewsletter.com/diabetes/product/foot-health-care/

The Ability of Your Kidneys and Pancreas Fail to Function Properly

- kidneys: https://healthylifestylenewsletter.com/diabetes/what-happens-if-type-2-diabetes-is-not-addressed-or-detected/
- diabetes management: https://healthylifestylenewsletter.com/diabetes/about/

Nerve Damage Risk Increases With Type 2 Diabetes

- Diabetic neuropathy: https://healthylifestylenewsletter.com/diabetes/product/diabetic-neuropathy/

Ensuing Vision Problems with Type 2 Diabetes

- none

Skin Issues as a Diabetic
diabetes management: https://healthylifestylenewsletter.com/diabetes/

Changes to the Reproductive Systems as a Diabetic

- none

Increased Risk of Dental Issues When Living with Diabetes

- none

The Emotional Well-Being at Risk

- none

Final Thoughts

- Hypoglycemia: https://healthylifestylenewsletter.com/diabetes/wp-content/uploads/improvedsqueezepage/index.html
- walking: https://www.amazon.com/gp/product/B078G424FB
- muscle builder: https://www.amazon.com/gp/product/B00XLOL52E
- low carb diet: https://www.amazon.com/gp/product/B00VIFY7WI
- high fat: https://www.amazon.com/gp/product/B07NQ2Z67X
- delicious and satisfying meals: https://healthylifestylenewsletter.com/diabetes/product/diets-for-diabetes/

About the Author

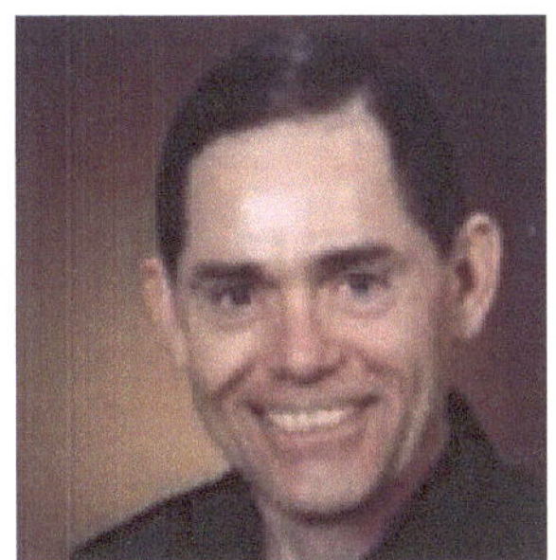

I have published over 125 books on Amazon for Kindle, CreateSpace and other publishing platforms.

While most of my books are on health and fitness in general, as I age (now 65) at the time of this writing) my topics of interest are geared toward aging baby boomers and older.

Besides my own writing, I also ghostwrite ebooks, books, reports, articles, blogs and do Kindle conversions for clients on a variety of topics.

Today my wife and I are retired from our careers and live in Gold Canyon, AZ. I now write as a retirement business where you'll find me happily sitting in my office typing away on my laptop as I work on my next book or ghostwriting project . . . that is if we are not traveling on a cruise ship - our new-found mode of travel.

www.ingramcontent.com/pod-product-compliance
Lightning Source LLC
Chambersburg PA
CBHW040048240726
48664CB00004B/1104

* 9 7 8 1 7 9 8 1 9 2 1 5 3 *